Just Power Walking
Essential Guide to Walking for Weight Loss

How Walking Can Help You Lose Weight

and Fat

Ann Vase

TABLE OF CONTENTS

Introduction

One of the keys to living a long healthy life is maintaining an active lifestyle and drinking plenty of water. Water may not be the sexy choice but, it help to shed the weight. Today, many people follow hectic schedules that leave little time for physical fitness activities. As a result, obesity has reached epidemic proportions in the world and heart disease and diabetes (two conditions linked to sedentary lifestyles) are on the rise. Indeed, the consequences of neglecting physical fitness activities can be felt in both the rising medical costs to treat these conditions and in higher mortality rates.

To their credit, many people have tried to combat this disturbing trend by joining gyms or health clubs. That said, gym memberships can be financially prohibitive for many and the routines quite monotonous for others. Statistics show that few people maintain gym-based physical fitness routines for prolonged periods of time.

Is there, then, a realistic and affordable way to incorporate exercise into a busy schedule that can add years to your life? The answer is yes. People are walking for fitness and studies find that it can have a significant impact on overall health.

Power walking is a great way to improve or maintain your overall health. Just 30 minutes every day can increase cardiovascular fitness, strengthen bones, reduce excess body fat, and boost muscle power and endurance. It can also reduce your risk of developing conditions such as heart disease, type 2 diabetes, osteoporosis and some cancers. Unlike some other forms of exercise, walking is free and doesn't require any special equipment or training.

Physical activity does not have to be vigorous or done for long periods in order to improve your health. A 2007 study of inactive women found that even a low level of exercise - around 75 minutes per week - improved their fitness levels significantly, when compared to a non-exercising group.

Power walking is low impact, requires minimal equipment, can be done at any time of day and can be performed at your own pace. You can get out and walk without worrying about the risks associated with some more vigorous forms of exercise. Walking is also a great form of physical activity for people who are overweight, elderly, or who haven't exercised in a long time.

Power walking for fun and fitness isn't limited to strolling by yourself around local neighborhood streets. There are various clubs, venues and strategies you can use to make walking an enjoyable and social part of your lifestyle.

How Walking Can Benefit You

Today

From strengthening bones to shedding pounds, researchers keep finding more and more health benefits from this simple activity. Need a reason to hit the trail or wander the pavement? Here are just a few impressive benefits of walking.

Aids Weight Loss. Walking is a great exercise and helps you lose weight. American scientists designed an experiment where obese patients walked together to their destinations in and around the city. After 8 weeks, their weight was checked, and more than 50% of the participants lost an average of 5 pounds. Therefore, it might be a good idea to start walking to and from your nearby destinations, instead of driving your car.

It helps you maintain a healthy weight. It may seem like a no-brainer, but regular walking can lead to weight loss because exercise burns calories. But with walking, the calories you burn depend more the distance you cover rather than your pace, according to Harvard Health. During a 15-year study, researchers found that people who walked gained significantly less weight than those who didn't and the more people walked, the less weight they gained.

It saves your brain. Walking keeps your mind sharp. In a University of California at San Francisco study, researchers measured the cognitive abilities of nearly 6,000 women age 65 and older. They tracked their physical activity for several years and found that age-related memory decline was lowest in the women who walked the most. Another study published in the December 2018 issue of Neurology shows that older adults who never exercise and already show signs of cognitive concerns can reverse cognitive decline (i.e. decision-making skills) in as little as six months just by walking.

It can help you live longer. Several studies have linked regular walking to longevity. A 2018 study found that walking can lower your risk of dying from cardiovascular disease. Another study in 2018 found that walking at a brisk pace seems to cut the risk of dying by 24 percent, while walking at an average pace reduces the risk by 20 percent. A study by the American Cancer Society found that even low levels of walking are linked with lower mortality.

Power walking strengthens bones and muscles. All those steps can keep your bones strong and ward off bone loss, fractures and osteoporosis. That back-and-forth movement also tones the muscles in your legs and abs. If you swing your arms when you walk, you can strengthen those arm muscles, too.

It eases joint pain. Walking protects your joints by lubricating them and strengthening the surrounding muscles that support them. Several studies also have shown that walking eases arthritis-related pain and if you walk enough, it might prevent arthritis from forming in the first place.

It boosts your mood. The more people walk each day, the more energetic they feel and the better their mood, according to a California State University study. Walking releases endorphins, which are chemicals that trigger positive feelings in the body.

It can reduce your breast cancer risk. An American Cancer Society study found that women who walked seven or more hours a week had a 14 percent lower risk of developing breast cancer than those who walked three hours or fewer per week.

Walking can help you sleep. An hour of walking and stretching, especially in the morning, can help you fall asleep and stay asleep.

It can reduce your risk of diabetes. Walking can help prevent diabetes or reduce its severity. Findings from the Harvard Nurses' Health Study suggest that walking briskly for 30 minutes daily reduces the risk of developing Type 2 diabetes by 30 percent.

It helps your heart. Walking does wonders for your heart and circulation, according to the Arthritis Foundation. It lowers your blood pressure, strengthens your heart, cuts your risk of stroke and wards off heart disease.

Getting Proper Shoes and Clothing

For Walking

Walking is a low-cost and effective form of exercise. However, the wrong type of shoe or walking action can cause foot or shin pain, blisters and injuries to soft tissue. Make sure your shoes are comfortable, with appropriate heel and arch supports. Take light, easy steps and make sure your heel touches down before your toes. Whenever possible, walk on grass rather than concrete to help absorb the impact. Familiarize yourself with what to wear and what to avoid before you start walking.

Shoes

When choosing walking shoes, it's important to know the basics of a walking shoe, as knowing this information will help you choose a shoe that will benefit both your foot health and improve your walking performance. Here are some basic tips and information for choosing a good pair of walking shoe.

The mechanics of walking shoe designs are geared towards helping the foot bear the stress of impact and balance the weight of the entire body during walking. If you're on your feet for long periods using inappropriate walking shoes, you might even experience unusual pain in your back or calves. The science of walking shoe design takes into account the different foot types to ensure maximum support and comfort for flat feet, normal feet, or high-arched feet. For each foot type, shoe designers add features to enhance efficiency, correct poor mechanics, protect the feet from injuries and to provide optimal stability. Shoes for walking for flat feet have medial posts or devices like the rollbar for greater stability and mechanical correction. These are often called stability or motion control shoes. Normal feet are best suited with neutral-cushioning and stability shoes which offer low-to-moderate stability with cushioning and higher flexibility. High-arched feet are better off with flexible, highly cushioned shoes for impact absorption.

Apart from comfort and overall support, walking shoes have extra added features to suit the needs of serious athletes, occasional walkers, and fitness walkers. Generally, your choice in walking shoes should have low and stable heels and generous toe room. When shopping for the best fitting walking shoes, focus on function rather than the form and it is to your advantage if you have different sets of walking shoes to allow for decompression after all that walking. Shoes have to take a break, too.

After your foot type, you should consider where you will be wearing your shoes. Will you be walking on smooth pavements or rough roads? Will you be walking on your treadmill? Are you on the heavy side? Take these things into consideration, too:

- Motion control shoes are for people with extra weight. This shoe type gives excellent support but has a thicker, more stable heel. These are typically heavier and less flexible.
- Stability shoes are for people with normal or average feet. These shoes have great combinations of cushioning and support.
- Cushioned shoes give extra comfort for people with high arches. High arches have minimal capacity for shock absorption, hence, extra cushion support is needed to protect the feet from injury.
- Race walking shoes are lightweight and can take on higher speeds but they are not as durable and offer less support and stability than other walking shoes.
- Outdoor walking and hiking shoes are sturdier than sneakers and offer superior traction and protection from the elements.

Your shoes should have a comfortable fit and should be flexible to allow for various walking motions. Ensure a good fit by buying shoes in the afternoon when your feet have swelled to its widest size. Also, test the shoes with sport socks on because these socks take up space. Consider mesh styles if your feet sweat too much. These are lighter and give more ventilation. For wet weather, walking footwear with waterproof-treated leather and synthetic uppers are perfect. With the right walking shoes, you can remain comfortable on your feet all day.

Socks

Choose high-tech fibers and avoid cotton. Your socks should be comfortable, and the modern running socks made from CoolMax or other high-tech fibers are preferable to cotton, which hold sweat next to the skin and allow blisters to form more quickly. Your walking socks should be made of a sweat-wicking fabric. They should be anatomically designed, rather than tube socks, so they stay in place at toe and heel.

Walking Pants

Denim is a bad walking choice. In hot weather, it is heavy and hot and holds sweat next to your skin. In wet weather, it soaks up rain like a sponge. If you end up wet from either sweat or rain, you may soon be chafed on your thighs and crotch. Instead, choose walking pants made from a sweat-wicking fabric.

Shirts

For your shoulders, even if you wear a good sunscreen, wearing a skin-baring tank top provides too much sun exposure. It all adds up over the years to age your skin and raise your risk of skin cancer. It's best to wear short sleeves as a sun safety measure. If you sweat while walking, you should invest in CoolMax or polypropylene shirts to wick the sweat away from the body.

Layers

Depending on your climate, dress in layers so you may remove a layer as you warm up while walking and put it back on if you feel cool. If you are warm when you start walking, you will soon be too hot. Start off feeling slightly cool. If you do not plan to walk up a sweat, a system can be as simple as a t-shirt, light sweater (wool or down), and windproof jacket which may also be waterproof. Unless you are walking in subfreezing temperatures, this is all you need. Add a hat, gloves or scarf for extra comfort.

How to Commit to a Walking Program

You want to walk, but how do you get yourself out the door or onto the treadmill? That's the toughest challenge many people face. If you are a natural couch potato, you face it every day. But you can learn ways to motivate yourself and get healthy exercise consistently.

Here are some tactics that I use to keep me motivated and inspired to work out:

Set goals: Nothing will motivate you more than trying to achieve a goal. Don't just say, "I want to lose 20 pounds this year." One thing I can tell you for sure is that 99% of people who set a weight goal never achieve it. Add more fun to it! Make yourself accountable. My wife has been trying to get active since we had our second child. Finally, I convinced her to sign up for a half-marathon. Once she did,

16

she never missed a run on her schedule, and most importantly, she now enjoys running.

So find a local 5k, a half or full marathon, or any active event, and sign up for it. If you like rock climbing, set a goal to summit a mountain! Start with a small goal or one that's difficult to even imagine as reachable, but do make a goal. As Nike so succinctly says: "Just do it!" I like to set a goal of a minimum of two big races during my season: one in the spring, and one in the fall. That way I am motivated and have something to look forward to throughout the year

Make It A Priority: Ask yourself: "How do I want to feel when I wake up in the morning? Would I rather be caught up on my favorite late-night TV show but wake up tired? Or, would I rather go to bed earlier so that I may rise refreshed and energized to get a workout in?" I really struggled initially when training for my first triathlon. I had no idea how to fit in my workouts into my already busy schedule, while simultaneously living up to my family, career, and home-owner expectations. However, it was very important to me, and I was highly motivated to find a doable solution. I was never a morning person but realized it was the only time I could get my workouts in. It wasn't easy at first, but slowly I got used to a new routine. Now, even on vacation days, by the time my wife and kids are awake, I am usually close, or already done with a long workout. You can always DVR the shows you like or watch them online.

Schedule A Regular Workout Time. Some of the most committed athletes work out very early in the morning. No one will schedule a meeting at 4 or 5am. It will be just you and the road, and no one will bother you. If mornings are hectic for you, then see what time of the day will work better for you and commit to it. Many athletes I know have early job commitments, so mornings are not an ideal time for workouts, yet they find time in the evening after their kids' bed time.

Wear a Pedometer or Fitness Band: Wearing a pedometer or fitness band can help motivate you to increase your activity. You can wear a device or start paying attention to the steps recorded by the pedometer app of your smartphone. Set your step goal at 6,000 to 10,000 per day, and find ways to add steps to your day.

Don't Waste Time: Make your workouts count. If you are out of the door, then get a good workout in. Don't stand around chatting with friends if your time is limited. Get there with a plan, and do it.

Keep It Simple: The more you complicate things, the higher the chance you will lose interest. You want to run? Get properly fitted running shoes and go out and run. No need to worry about ideal running gear, compression garnet, heart rate monitor, finding the latest and greatest gadget advertised in fitness magazines, or reading about

19

and searching online for the ultimate training program. Just start running, and you'll figure out the rest later. You want to eat healthy? Then ditch all the diet books and follow the "common sense" diet. There is no magic diet formula out there, no 30-day miraculous transformation. Eat healthy and get most of your daily calories from fruit, vegetables, raw nuts, and good protein. Avoid processed food, processed sugar, or any type of sweeteners. Read labels, and if you can't pronounce it, don't eat it.

Surround Yourself With Active People: Get to know active people at your local gym. Join a masters swim group or ask your local bike shop or running store about group rides or weekly group runs. You will make a lot of friends that will keep you motivated and from whom you will learn. You can also find and join an active group on many of the social networking sites

Use Social Media: Many like to use social media such as Facebook, Twitter, or more fitness specific ones such as Runkeeper, Strava, DailyMile to post their workouts. Telling your followers about your workouts makes you feel accountable. Also, many find motivation from reading others' workouts.

Mix It Up: By nature, we need change to keep motivated. If you keep doing the same thing over and over again, you will get burned out. Start running trails or different routes, or try to challenge yourself differently in a workout. Try different sports. If you belong to a gym, look at the group workouts they offer and try something different. It's a great way to challenge yourself and stay motivated at the same time.

Reward Yourself: Buy New Gear. When training for long hours, one of the methods that have been proven to keep athletes motivated is new gear. The smell of new running shoes or that coveted GPS watch can get you going. Even loading new music into the iPod can spark your workouts. So start thinking of yourself as an athlete and not a spectator. Set a goal, mark it on your calendar, and have fun with it. You'll quickly realize the benefits of better health, more energy, and more happiness.

Benefit Of Taking 10,000 Steps For

Optimal Fat Loss

It's been claimed that individuals can lose a pound of fat a week just by taking 10,000 steps a day because of the potential to burn 3,500 calories from walking. As a general rule of thumb, a pound of fat contains around 3,500 calories. If you create an average caloric deficit of 500 calories over a 7-day period, that's equal to 3,500 calories: good for a pound of weight loss per week.

Unfortunately, that 10,000/day = 3,500 calories/week calculation is based on estimations of a specific body type, so this may not apply to you. To understand why, let's break this claim down.

Weight

Any estimation of how many calories you burn from an exercise like walking or running is dependent on how heavy you are. Heavier people on average use more energy to move than lighter people. Most rough estimates revolve around 100 calories burned per mile for a 180-pound person. And 10,000 steps is roughly 5 miles. So assuming you weigh 180 pounds then yes, by simple mathematics, 100 calories x 5 miles equals 500 calories. Over the course of a week that becomes 3,500 calories. But if you're lighter or heavier, you will burn less/more calories while taking the same number of steps or walking the same distance.

If you were 120-pounds, in that same mile you would only burn 60 calories. Calculate that over the course of a week and that only becomes 2,100 calories, meaning that you are 1,400 calories short of reaching that 3,500 calorie goal.

Walking Speed and Distance

Even if you happen to be at that 180-pound range, the calories you burn from walking depend on the intensity, or speed, of your walk. The average walking speed is about 3 miles per hour, and according to the Mayo Clinic, the number of calories you'll burn depends on your walking speed.

For a 180-pound person, a leisurely 30-minute walk at 2 mph yields a burn of 102 calories, but walk at a more moderate intensity (3.5 mph) in the same 30-minute walk and the calorie burn increases by 54% to 157 calories.

Why? It's simple: the faster the pace the greater your heart rate, and the more you can burn covering the same distance. The sources that suggest you can average weight loss of a pound a week from walking typically assume you walk at the pace necessary to cover the estimated 5-mile distance. If you deviate from either of the above conditions, your results may differ. But even if you reach 10,000 steps, all of that effort can almost entirely be irrelevant if you aren't careful: weight loss from walking largely assumes your caloric intake stays the stable.

You Can't Walk Away From Your Diet

There's no doubt that walking leads to more calories burned throughout the day. However, without understanding your calorie net caloric balance, walking 10,000 steps, 15,000 steps, or even 20,000 steps a day might not be enough to cause any meaningful fat loss or improvements to body composition.

In order to achieve fat loss, you need to burn more calories than you get from your food. That's called a caloric deficit. For example, let's say that you need 1,800 calories a day to maintain your current body weight, but you have a daily caloric intake of 2300. Assuming your 10,000 steps equal 500 calories burned (which, as shown above, is far from guaranteed), you'd only be bringing yourself to a net caloric balance of zero, meaning the 10,000 steps you are taking are only help you maintain your current weight, not lose the weight.

There's no question that there are enormous health benefits to increasing your activity level through moderate exercises like walking, even if they don't necessarily lead to weight loss. A 2010 study has shown that walking more has a whole host of positive health benefits, including improved cardiovascular health, cholesterol level, fitness ability and many other variables that contribute towards healthy living. In another study cited by the American Heart Association, researchers found that a regular brisk walk can lower the risk of developing high blood pressure, high cholesterol, and diabetes.

It's safe to say that everyone reading this ebook now could likely benefit from adopting a healthy habit like walking. But if weight loss is your mission, it's important that you understand how weight loss occurs so you can set appropriate goals to help you achieve it, and that includes putting goals like walking 10,000 steps a day into context.

Weight loss occurs when you're in a caloric deficit. If your calories in/out are in balance, you can't expect much change. You've got to get out of balance for change to happen, and generally, the easiest way to do that is by increasing exercise and decreasing your caloric intake.

Setting and achieving a daily goal like 10,000 steps can be a great way to increase your activity level and create a healthy lifestyle. You can add walking as a warm-up before a strength training workout, or it can be a workout by itself. But before you set any fitness goal like walking 10,000 steps, take a minute to understand what you're embarking on. Remember the old Chinese proverb, "A journey of a thousand miles begins with a single step." Make sure each step, from the first to the 10,000th to the 100,000th has a purpose.

Walking On A Treadmill Vs.

Outside

Because time is often a factor, many people wonder which cardiovascular activity will give them the best workout for their effort. Walking outdoors is available to most people, though weather and location can be a limiting factor in some situations. Walking on a treadmill requires access to a treadmill, either in your home or at a fitness club. Though both workouts offer the benefits of walking, there are distinct advantages and disadvantages to each.

Walking is an accessible activity: most everyone can do it. All you need is a pair of comfortable shoes. Because of this, walking is an attractive workout option for many individuals. Walking is also a low-impact activity; stress on the joints of the legs, hips and back is minimal. Those new to exercise are often attracted to walking because it does not require an additional skill or significant equipment. Individuals recovering from injury can also reap the benefits of exercise without less risk of reinjuring themselves.

Benefits of Walking Outside

Walking outdoors is simple exercise. Most people have access to sidewalks or local trails, making outdoor walking convenient and affordable. A brisk, 30-minute walk in your neighborhood is an excellent way to improve cardiovascular fitness. The varied terrain, combined with proprioception (the neural-muscular response to outside stimuli), keeps the brain engaged in the workout as well. Because the walking surface--whether it be concrete, grass or a trail--is slightly modified with each step, the walker must integrate these changing perceptions to maintain a comfortable stride.

Benefits of a Treadmill

A treadmill offers a variety of options to simulate outdoor walking when outdoor walking may be unavailable. Treadmills allow you to customize your workout: you can choose to walk hills on a treadmill, even if you live in a relatively flat area. Having access to a treadmill, either at home or at a fitness club, allows you to walk when extreme weather prohibits walking outdoors. The surface of a treadmill is more forgiving than a concrete or asphalt sidewalk, putting less strain on your joints.

Comparison

The surface of a treadmill is consistent, making it a great choice for injured walkers or even those new to exercise. On the other hand, a treadmill does not engage the brain's sensory receptors as completely as outdoor walking does. Additionally, you must overcome air resistance while walking outdoors. A high-quality treadmill is an expensive purchase. A gym membership may also be prohibitively expensive for some individuals. Walking outdoors is free, provided you can find a safe place to walk. For most people, however, the most important factor when choosing an exercise type is consistency. You will reap the benefits of exercise whether you walk outdoors or on a treadmill; the key is to walk regularly and briskly.

The type of walking workout you choose should be based upon your own fitness goals. If you begin walking as a form of training for an outdoor event, such as a hike, you should try to mimic the event's conditions as much as possible. At the same time, outdoor walking is better for those who do not have access to a treadmill or enjoy changes in weather and natural terrain. Treadmill walking, on the other hand, is better for those who want to customize and track their workouts using a machine.

Nutritional Protocol for Walking

The simple fact is that all exercise uses the body's stored energy, no matter what intensity. If these stores are not replaced, then over time energy will run low and performance will decline. As we know, the energy that foods contain is expressed in calories. Although every calorie provides the same amount of energy, the way in which the body breaks down a calorie from a carbohydrate, protein or fat differs vastly. That's why it's vital to consider different energy sources when fuelling for walks.

Carbohydrate is to exercise what petrol is to a car. It's the body's preferred energy source, as it's more readily converted to energy than fat. We have a small amount of carbohydrate circulating in the blood as glucose, with most stored in the muscles and liver as glycogen. This is very limited compared to the body's fat stores, which could theoretically provide enough energy to power a walker for 1,300kms.

In simple terms, when glycogen stores deplete, your muscles and brain run out of fuel, making us feel exhausted and drained. The good news for hikers is that due to slower pace and lower overall heart rate, it is a lot longer before you hit that 'wall', since the body also uses fat stores alongside carbohydrate for energy. Fat oxidation is not fast enough to provide energy during high intensity exercise but is fine for moderate walking speed.

Protein has a different role. There is no evidence that consuming protein during exercise improves performance, but since it takes longer to digest than carbohydrate, the advantage of eating protein on a walk is that it will keep you full for longer, as well as providing a savoury taste change to carbohydrate.

So do we really need to worry about what we eat when out walking? It seems like the body looks after itself. Unfortunately, this is not the case.

Fuelling requirements when walking will differ greatly depending on factors such as length of walk, altitude, temperature and weight carried. The type of carbohydrates that are needed will also differ at various stages of your walk.

Nutrition

Carbohydrate-rich foods come in various forms, which can be classified by the Glycaemic Index (GI). This measures how much a food increases blood sugar levels. Low GI foods that don't greatly boost blood sugar such as oats, seeded bread, pasta, yoghurt and some fruits offer a sustained release of energy over time. They are good to eat pre- hike or during a lunch stop, as they keep you fuller for longer.

However, there are times when your body may benefit from a quick release of energy through high GI foods, such as ripe bananas, a white bread jam sandwich, jelly babies or energy bars. These are perfect for energy 'on the go', when blood sugar levels have dropped and instant, easily absorbed energy is needed.

Hydration

As well as nutrition, hydration is vital to performance. If you don't drink enough, especially in hot conditions or at altitude, your performance will decline significantly. Severe dehydration can be dangerous, as it can mean you become confused and disorientated, so be aware of the early signs, such as headaches. How much fluid you need depends on the duration of your walk, air temperature, altitude and how much you sweat. The key is to make sure you start your hike well-hydrated. If your urine is clear, you can be reassured that this is the case.

When the weather is brutally hot and you are likely to sweat a lot, consider taking sports drinks or tabs to replace lost electrolytes. The balance of electrolytes in the body affects and regulates hydration as well as being important to nerve and muscle function. Electrolyte drinks containing sodium and potassium salts help to replenish the body's electrolytes.

There is no need to over drink, just be guided by your body and drink according to thirst. In hotter environments a more structured approach may be needed, such as drinking 100-250mls every 15 minutes, but the best advice is to stay vigilant and listen to your body.

Walking Equipment To Make Your Walks More Effective

What walking equipment do you really need? Truthfully, you don't need much. That is why I love this sport; there isn't any expensive gear to buy.

However, the gear that I do recommended on this page will make exercising more comfortable and your life a little easier by tracking how much distance you've logged and how many calories you've burned.

Pedometer. A pedometer will count your daily steps, total mileage and calories burned. This is a very handy device to keep track of your progress. You can buy for as little as $15. Read this article on the best pedometers to ensure you are buying an accurate and affordable pedometer.

A Good Pair Of Walking Shoes. This is probably the most important gear you need. A well fitting pair of shoes can prevent many kinds of injuries and sprains to your feet, legs and back. Here are my tips for finding the perfect fitting pair of shoes.

Walking Music. Fitness walking and music that you enjoy will give you a boost of energy. There is nothing like hearing your favorite songs to get you moving. Learn more about which walking music is best for your fitness level in this article.

Fitness Walking Books. It's great to have a book on hand when you can't logon to The-Fitness-Walking-Guide.com   :)   Here   are   my recommendations for fitness walking books.

Walking DVDs or Walking Videos. For those days when you can't leave the house, pop in a walking DVD or video and get your walking workout done in your bedroom or living room. See my recommendations for fitness walking DVDs and videos

Hydration Belt/Waist Pack. Ever wonder where to stash your keys, cell phone and water bottle while walking? A hydration belt is a hands-free way to carry all of these items. Here are my recommendations for the most useful and affordable Hydration Belts.

Walking Hand Weights. The use of walking hand weights will add variety and challenge to your walking routine.

They will help build muscle in your triceps, biceps, chest, shoulders and core. They will also increase the intensity of your cardio workout, which will burn even more calories during your walk. Read this article on my recommendations for walking hand weights.

There are a lot of new fitness gadgets that make using technology very easy to monitor your walking and weight loss goals. Items like the Jawbone or Fitbit exercise trackers can help you keep track of how active you are, how well you sleep and how many calories you consume. Here is a fascinating article about how we are beginning to integrate such technology into our lives. Now you have recommendations for the walking equipment you need to get the most out of each and every walk. You'll find your walks safer and more enjoyable too.

Join Walking Clubs

Many people look upon their leisure time as an opportunity to meet new people other than their close friends and work colleagues in an effort to forge new friendships and to get a different perspective on life and exchange views and ideas. Walkers are no different in this regard. Additionally, some walkers feel more secure when out walking with a group especially if they're hiking in unfamiliar and sometimes challenging terrain. Usually in these situations, the group will have a trip leader and their help and support can be invaluable and often gives walkers more confidence to tackle walks which they might otherwise have shied away from on their own. By overcoming these hurdles with the help of more experienced walkers, it can often increase a walker's self-confidence and instils in them a belief that they can face other subsequent challenges confidently. There are also plenty of walkers who prefer to join a walking club as group participation usually means that their voice will be heard regarding important matters to hiking in general. For example, the 'freedom to roam' only came about with the help of a vast number of walkers combining forces, assisted by other organizations, to campaign for the right to have access to public or privately owned land for recreation and exercise. Similarly, groups of organized walkers belonging to a hiking club are better placed to campaign to protect landscapes, the public footpath network, long distance walking routes and our National Parks. And, if you have a particular empathy with a specific area of environmental or conservational interest, you can be sure that there is probably a walking club or organization which is sympathetic to the same cause.

A walking club will consist of walkers of all ages and social backgrounds. One of the benefits of joining a walking club will be that you'll get to meet a whole variety of people many of whom you might not otherwise have come across in your normal everyday life so the social aspect of being a member of a club can broaden your horizons. Also, if you're a beginner, you'll not feel the odd one out as there are bound to be other beginners walking with you which, in itself, creates a common bond likely to result in new friendships. Likewise, there will also be highly experienced walkers who can offer you advice and some useful hiking tips. They'll also be able to tell you the best places to buy gear and many clubs will often have some kind of affiliation with certain youth hostels etc. and outdoor retailers where you'll benefit from cheaper rates and prices. A walking club will also give you the opportunity to venture out to different walking locations and to visit places you may not otherwise have visited. One of the great attractions about hiking is that you will experience something new and different every time you head out on a walk and never more so than when you're walking along different trails in other areas of the county or, indeed, even further afield. And, unlike non-organised groups which can create a problem if there are walkers of different levels of fitness and expertise, many hiking clubs often have separate walks each weekend to suit different levels of ability. For example, Group A may be the most advanced group and may end up going for a 20 mile hike on difficult, hilly terrain whilst Group D may be for 'newbies' who are just starting out with an 8 mile hike on flat marshland.

Walking Mistakes To Avoid

Beginners

You've been walking nearly your entire life, so surely you know a thing or two about putting one foot in front of the other, right? Not so much. Walking for fitness isn't the same as taking a walk in the park. In order to stay injury-free while reaping all of the disease-fighting, fat-blasting, and mood-boosting benefits of walking, it's important to pay attention to what your body is doing from head to toe. To make sure you're striding right, beware of these 10 common pitfalls:

Mistake: Thinking it's all about your lower body

Your feet, ankles, and legs are propelling you forward, but the rest of your body - especially your core - shouldn't just be along for the ride. "When your core muscles are strong and activated while walking, they take some of the pressure off your feet and toes, which reduces your risk of overuse injuries. While walking, draw your belly button toward your spine, being careful not to grip the muscles. Lean your torso slightly forward to keep your core muscles engaged - leaning back releases them.

Mistake: Walking with flimsy arms

Allowing your arms to just hang there creates more work for your body and slows your pace. Instead, bend your elbows to 90° and relax your shoulders. As you walk, move your arms naturally in opposition with your feet so that when your left foot is forward, your right arm is forward and vice versa. In addition to making you more efficient, bending your arms increases calorie burn and toning compared to letting them go limp.

Mistake: Focusing on what you wear to work out, but not on what you wear to work

Ballet flats seem like a better choice than heels, but if you have flat arches they don't provide enough support and if you have high arches they allow your arch to collapse every time you take a step. Over time, these issues can cause plantar fasciitis, a common and painful condition in which the band of tissue that runs across the bottom of your foot becomes inflamed. An injury like that can derail your walking program no matter how great your walking shoes may be. Opt for a wedge or low heel, which provide more support than completely flat kicks.

Mistake: Letting your mind wander the entire time

If you always let your mind go free on your walks, you're missing an opportunity to strengthen your mind-body connection. Instead, periodically check in with what the different parts of your body are doing: Are your shoulders relaxed? Are your elbows bent? Is your core engaged? And so on.

And, like yoga, pay attention to your breathing. A very common mistake is that people don't breathe enough while walking. For every breath out, take about 3 to 4 steps, and for every breath in take about 2 steps. Not only will you keep your mind focused and calm, but you'll send your breath deeper into your lungs and give yourself more energy.

Mistake: Sticking to the treadmill

For an even more zen-like experience (while torching calories and challenging your cardiovascular fitness), head for greener spaces. Several recent studies show that people who exercise outdoors experience less tension, depression, and fatigue than those who walk indoors.

Mistake: Avoiding hills

Heading for the hills isn't always possible, but if you can find them, climb them. Huffing an incline strengthens muscles that may otherwise get neglected when walking on flatter surfaces. A study found that when walking at an incline, the activity in muscles such as your quadriceps, glutes, calf, knee, and ankle increase by up to 635% which of course means more toning power. You can get the same benefits by increasing a treadmill's incline about 9 degrees or regularly adding stairs to your walking routine.

Mistake: Going too easy on yourself

All walking is not created equal: Strolling is better than sitting, but to score walking's cardio, strength, and fat-burning effects, you need to push yourself a little harder. If you ask a runner what their one-mile pace is she'll probably know it, but many walkers don't. But you should! When walking for fitness, you should aim for a 15-minute mile. Not there yet? No worries. Simply work toward that goal. Keep track of your pace with a free app, such as Strava or MapMyWalk, or a fitness-tracking device, or simply use a stopwatch or pedometer.

Please Set Walking Goals

Made in the USA
Coppell, TX
06 June 2020

27031058R00032